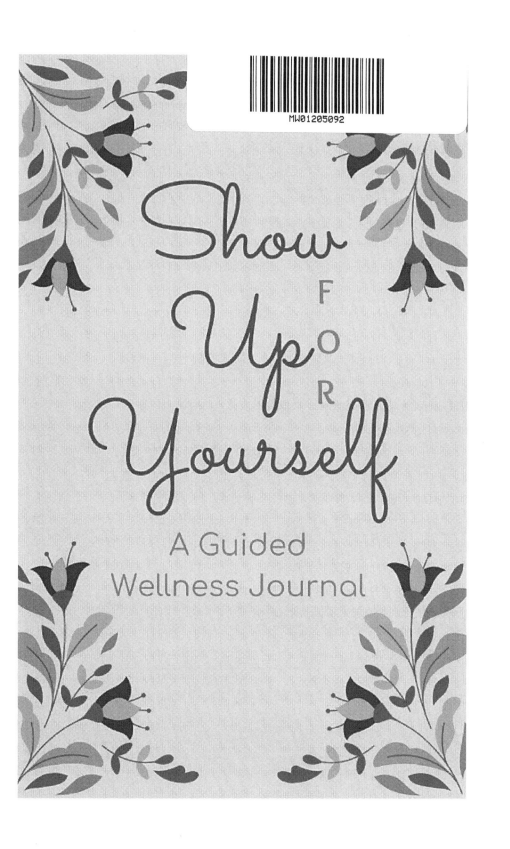

Show
F
O
R
Up
Yourself

A Guided
Wellness Journal

Author: PersoNell Wellness

Exterior and Interior design by Chaunell Walker.

Published by PersoNell Wellness.

Manufactured in United States of America.

Quote Credits: Chaunell Walker, R.S. Grey, Robert Louis Stevenson, Josh Billings, scriptures are from The King James Version, *Holy Bible*, New Living Translation, copyright © 1996, 2004, 2015 by Tyndale House Foundation.

Introduction

This jumpstart journal will serve as your guide to the best version of you yet! It is designed to help you navigate a 21-day wellness journey.

You've shown up for everyone else throughout your life. Now, it is time to show up for one of the most important people on earth - YOU!

Everywhere we turn now-a-days there is mention of Wellness, but do we really understand what it is, or for that matter, how we start to achieve it?

What is Wellness and how do I achieve it?

I am glad you asked, Friend. Wellness is a state of being healthy in mind, body, spirit, and emotions as the result of deliberate healthy lifestyle choices.

A focus on mind, body, spirit, and emotions is a holistic approach to wellness - the fundamentals. However, wellness may also include other factors such as a person's social, environmental, and financial lifestyle choices. This journal will address the fundamentals.

Many experts agree that 21 consecutive days is an ideal start to form a habit pattern. The objective is to use this journal (for 21 days straight) to form healthy habits that become a part of your lifestyle, therefore, achieving personal wellness.

About This Journal

The "Show Up FOR Yourself" journal is a powerful tool for habit transformation, mindfulness, inspiration, and accountability.

Each day of your 21-day wellness journey, you will find the following prompt titles:

- ✓ Wellness Tracker
- ✓ Mood Check-in
- ✓ Mindfulness
- ✓ I'm Just Sayin' (for daily thoughts)

Additionally, you will find these prompt titles:

- ✓ This Week (to set the tone for the week)
- ✓ Mindset Matters
- ✓ You Did It!
- ✓ Growth
- ✓ Changes?
- ✓ What's Next?
- ✓ Follow-up
- ✓ Notes & Doodles (for notes, doodle drawings, stickers, reminders, etc.)

Let the prompts guide you to build healthy habits, set goals, identify triggers, take action, track progress, and reflect, but most of all – to Show. Up. For. Yourself.

Feel free to apply your new healthy habits to other areas of your life. Embrace change, be honest with yourself, and have fun. You deserve to be happy and healthy!

This Week

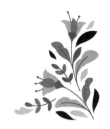

What mindset do you want to begin the week with?

- o Realistic
- o Honest
- o Fair
- o This is gonna be great!
- o I can't wait to tell everyone about my progress!
- o Diligent & Consistent
- o Eh, we'll see what happens.
- o Maybe this'll work. Won't know until I try.
- o This probably won't work.
- o Negativity will NOT live here, in Jesus' name!
- o Other (in your own words): ....
  ....
  ....

What are your intensions and expectations for this week?

....
....
....
....
....
....
....
....
....
....
....
....

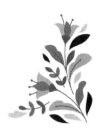

Mindset Matters

Your mindset will play a crucial part in your success. How will you apply this week's mindset to the following:

Mental Health ....
....

Physical Health ....
....

Spiritual Health ....
....

Emotional Health ....
....

Financial Health ....
....

Social Health ....
....

Environmental Health ....
....

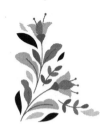 

Wellness Tracker

Date: ....

FOCUS	HOW I'M SHOWING UP FOR MYSELF
NUTRITION	
HYDRATION	
EXERCISE	
SLEEP	
DE-STRESS	
MY SPIRIT	
MY MIND	

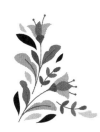

Mood Check-in

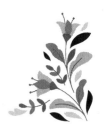

Checkmark the box that best describes how you feel.

TODAY	:) Happy Content	:| Blah Neutral	:(Sad Sick	Stressed Tired	Angry Annoyed
START OF DAY					
MID-DAY					
END OF DAY					

I NEED: ....

I FEEL THIS WAY BECAUSE: ....
....
....
....

PRAYER FOR THE DAY: ....
....
....
....
....
....

Mindfulness

POSITIVITY

I AM GRATEFUL FOR:
-
-
-
-

SMALL STEPS LEAD TO BIG RESULTS.

Do not despise these small beginnings, for the Lord rejoices to see the work begin.
(Zechariah 4:10 NLT)

LOOKING FORWARD TO:

....
....
....
....

ELIMINATE NEGATIVE SELF-TALK

TO DO:
-
-
-
-

SAY IT LOUD, I AM...
-
-
-
-

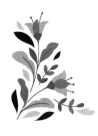

I'm Just Sayin'

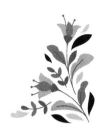

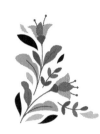

Wellness Tracker

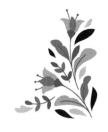

Date: ....

FOCUS	HOW I'M SHOWING UP FOR MYSELF
NUTRITION	
HYDRATION	
EXERCISE	
SLEEP	
DE-STRESS	
MY SPIRIT	
MY MIND	

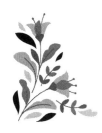
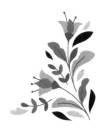

Mood Check-in

Checkmark the box that best describes how you feel.

TODAY	🙂 Happy Content	😐 Blah Neutral	🙁 Sad Sick	😟 Stressed Tired	😠 Angry Annoyed
START OF DAY					
MID-DAY					
END OF DAY					

I NEED: ....

I FEEL THIS WAY BECAUSE: ....
....
....
....

PRAYER FOR THE DAY: ....
....
....
....
....
....

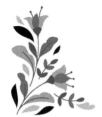
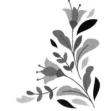

Mindfulness

POSITIVITY

YOUR BODY IS
THE GARDEN.

YOUR WILL IS
THE GARDENER.

ELIMINATE
NEGATIVE
SELF-TALK

I AM GRATEFUL FOR:

-
-
-
-

> *And you shall be like a watered garden, like a spring of water, whose waters fail not.*
> *(Isaiah 58:11 KJV)*

LOOKING FORWARD TO:

....
....
....
....

TO DO:

-
-
-
-

SAY IT LOUD, I AM...

-
-
-
-

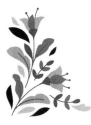
I'm Just Sayin'
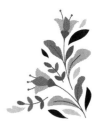

 # Wellness Tracker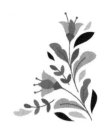

Date: ....

FOCUS	HOW I'M SHOWING UP FOR MYSELF
NUTRITION	
HYDRATION	
EXERCISE	
SLEEP	
DE-STRESS	
MY SPIRIT	
MY MIND	

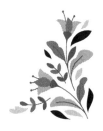

Mood Check-in

Checkmark the box that best describes how you feel.

TODAY	:) Happy Content	:| Blah Neutral	:(Sad Sick	Stressed Tired	Angry Annoyed
START OF DAY					
MID-DAY					
END OF DAY					

I NEED: ....

I FEEL THIS WAY BECAUSE: ....
....
....
....

PRAYER FOR THE DAY: ....
....
....
....
....
....

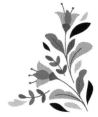

Mindfulness

POSITIVITY

DON'T STOP UNTIL YOU'RE PROUD.

ELIMINATE NEGATIVE SELF-TALK

I AM GRATEFUL FOR:

- ▪
- ▪
- ▪
- ▪

> *And let us not grow weary in well doing: for in due season we shall reap, if we faint not.*
> *(Galatians 6:9 KJV)*

LOOKING FORWARD TO:

....
....
....
....

TO DO:

- ▪
- ▪
- ▪
- ▪

SAY IT LOUD, I AM...

- ▪
- ▪
- ▪
- ▪

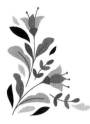
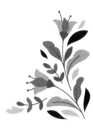

I'm Just Sayin'

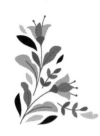
Wellness Tracker
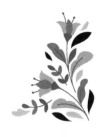

Date: ....

FOCUS	HOW I'M SHOWING UP FOR MYSELF
NUTRITION	
HYDRATION	
EXERCISE	
SLEEP	
DE-STRESS	
MY SPIRIT	
MY MIND	

Mood Check-in

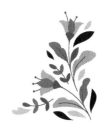

Checkmark the box that best describes how you feel.

TODAY	:) Happy Content	:| Blah Neutral	:(Sad Sick	Stressed Tired	Angry Annoyed
START OF DAY					
MID-DAY					
END OF DAY					

I NEED: ....

I FEEL THIS WAY BECAUSE: ....
....
....
....

PRAYER FOR THE DAY: ....
....
....
....
....

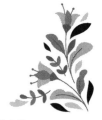

Mindfulness

POSITIVITY

I AM GRATEFUL FOR:

-
-
-
-

DON'T JUDGE EACH DAY BY THE HARVEST YOU REAP BUT BY THE SEEDS THAT YOU PLANT.

> I planted the seed in your hearts, and Apollos watered it, but it was God who made it grow.
> (1 Corinthians 3:6 NLT)

LOOKING FORWARD TO:

....
....
....
....

ELIMINATE NEGATIVE SELF-TALK

TO DO:

-
-
-

SAY IT LOUD, I AM...

-
-
-
-

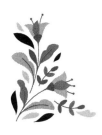
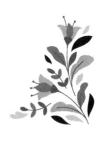

I'm Just Sayin'

Wellness Tracker

Date: ....

FOCUS	HOW I'M SHOWING UP FOR MYSELF
NUTRITION	
HYDRATION	
EXERCISE	
SLEEP	
DE-STRESS	
MY SPIRIT	
MY MIND	

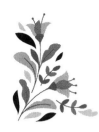

Mood Check-in

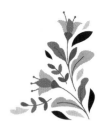

Checkmark the box that best describes how you feel.

TODAY	🙂 Happy Content	😐 Blah Neutral	🙁 Sad Sick	😟 Stressed Tired	😠 Angry Annoyed
START OF DAY					
MID-DAY					
END OF DAY					

I NEED: ....

I FEEL THIS WAY BECAUSE: ....

....

....

....

PRAYER FOR THE DAY: ....

....

....

....

....

....

Mindfulness

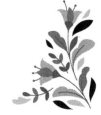

POSITIVITY

I AM GRATEFUL FOR:

-
-
-

SMILE!

IT INCREASES

YOUR FACE

VALUE.

> *A cheerful look brings joy to the heart; good news makes for good health. (Proverbs 15:30 NLT)*

LOOKING FORWARD TO:

....

....

....

....

TO DO:

-
-
-

ELIMINATE

NEGATIVE

SELF-TALK

SAY IT LOUD, I AM...

-
-
-

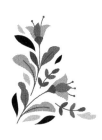
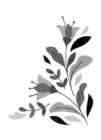

I'm Just Sayin'

Wellness Tracker

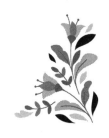

Date: ....

FOCUS	HOW I'M SHOWING UP FOR MYSELF
NUTRITION	
HYDRATION	
EXERCISE	
SLEEP	
DE-STRESS	
MY SPIRIT	
MY MIND	

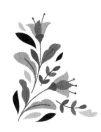

Mood Check-in

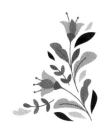

Checkmark the box that best describes how you feel.

TODAY	🙂 Happy Content	😐 Blah Neutral	🙁 Sad Sick	😟 Stressed Tired	😠 Angry Annoyed
START OF DAY					
MID-DAY					
END OF DAY					

I NEED: ....

I FEEL THIS WAY BECAUSE: ....
....
....
....

PRAYER FOR THE DAY: ....
....
....
....
....
....

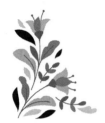 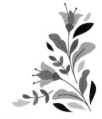

Mindfulness

POSITIVITY

I AM GRATEFUL FOR:

-
-
-
-

YOU KNOW WHAT'S SEXY?

WHOLENESS.

> But my God shall supply all your need according to His riches in glory by Christ Jesus.
> (Philippians 4:19 KJV)

LOOKING FORWARD TO:

....
....
....
....

ELIMINATE NEGATIVE SELF-TALK

TO DO:

-
-
-
-

SAY IT LOUD, I AM...

-
-
-
-

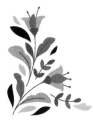

I'm Just Sayin'

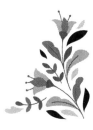

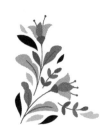
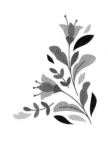

Wellness Tracker

Date: ....

FOCUS	HOW I'M SHOWING UP FOR MYSELF
NUTRITION	
HYDRATION	
EXERCISE	
SLEEP	
DE-STRESS	
MY SPIRIT	
MY MIND	

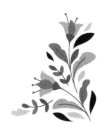

Mood Check-in

Checkmark the box that best describes how you feel.

TODAY	🙂 Happy Content	😐 Blah Neutral	🙁 Sad Sick	😟 Stressed Tired	😠 Angry Annoyed
START OF DAY					
MID-DAY					
END OF DAY					

I NEED: ....

I FEEL THIS WAY BECAUSE: ....
....
....
....

PRAYER FOR THE DAY: ....
....
....
....
....
....

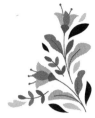

Mindfulness

POSITIVITY

I AM GRATEFUL FOR:

-
-
-

NO IS A COMPLETE SENTENCE.

> I'm not trying to win the approval of people, but of God. If pleasing people were my goal, I would not be Christ's servant.
> (Galatians 1:10 NLT)

LOOKING FORWARD TO:

....
....
....
....

ELIMINATE NEGATIVE SELF-TALK

TO DO:

-
-
-

SAY IT LOUD, I AM...

-
-
-

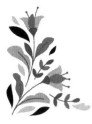
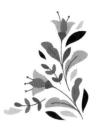

I'm Just Sayin'

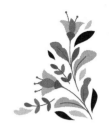

This Week

What mindset do you want to begin the week with?

- o Realistic
- o Honest
- o Fair
- o This is gonna be great!
- o I can't wait to tell everyone about my progress!
- o Diligent & Consistent
- o Eh, we'll see what happens.
- o Maybe this'll work. Won't know until I try.
- o This probably won't work.
- o Negativity will NOT live here, in Jesus' name!
- o Other (in your own words): ....
  ....
  ....

What are your intensions and expectations for this week?

....
....
....
....
....
....
....
....
....
....
....
....

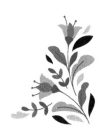

Mindset Matters

Your mindset will play a crucial part in your success. How will you apply this week's mindset to the following?

Mental Health ....
....

Physical Health ....
....

Spiritual Health ....
....

Emotional Health ....
....

Financial Health ....
....

Social Health ....
....

Environmental Health ....
....

Wellness Tracker

Date: ....

FOCUS	HOW I'M SHOWING UP FOR MYSELF
NUTRITION	
HYDRATION	
EXERCISE	
SLEEP	
DE-STRESS	
MY SPIRIT	
MY MIND	

Mood Check-in
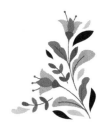

Checkmark the box that best describes how you feel.

TODAY	☺ Happy Content	😐 Blah Neutral	☹ Sad Sick	😟 Stressed Tired	😠 Angry Annoyed
START OF DAY					
MID-DAY					
END OF DAY					

I NEED: ....

I FEEL THIS WAY BECAUSE: ....
....
....
....

PRAYER FOR THE DAY: ....
....
....
....
....

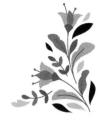

Mindfulness

POSITIVITY

YOU ARE CLOSER THAN EVER TO WHERE YOU WANT TO BE.

ELIMINATE NEGATIVE SELF-TALK

I AM GRATEFUL FOR:

-
-
-

> But as for you, be strong and courageous, for your work will be rewarded.
> (2 Chronicles 15:7 NLT)

LOOKING FORWARD TO:

....
....
....
....

TO DO:

-
-
-

SAY IT LOUD, I AM...

-
-
-

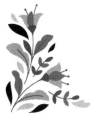
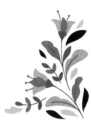

I'm Just Sayin'

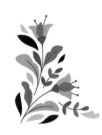

Wellness Tracker

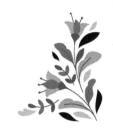

Date: ....

FOCUS	HOW I'M SHOWING UP FOR MYSELF
NUTRITION	
HYDRATION	
EXERCISE	
SLEEP	
DE-STRESS	
MY SPIRIT	
MY MIND	

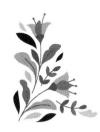

Mood Check-in

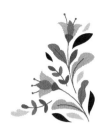

Checkmark the box that best describes how you feel.

TODAY	🙂 Happy Content	😐 Blah Neutral	🙁 Sad Sick	😟 Stressed Tired	😠 Angry Annoyed
START OF DAY					
MID-DAY					
END OF DAY					

I NEED: ....

I FEEL THIS WAY BECAUSE: ....
....
....
....

PRAYER FOR THE DAY: ....
....
....
....
....
....

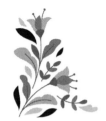
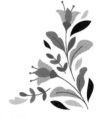

Mindfulness

POSITIVITY

TODAY, INHALE CONFIDENCE & EXHALE DOUBT.

I AM GRATEFUL FOR:

-
-
-

Blessed are those who trust in the LORD and have made the LORD their hope and confidence.
(Jeremiah 17:7 NLT)

LOOKING FORWARD TO:

....
....
....
....

TO DO:

-
-
-
-

ELIMINATE NEGATIVE SELF-TALK

SAY IT LOUD, I AM...

-
-
-
-

I'm Just Sayin'
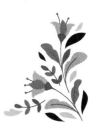

Wellness Tracker

Date: ....

FOCUS	HOW I'M SHOWING UP FOR MYSELF
NUTRITION	
HYDRATION	
EXERCISE	
SLEEP	
DE-STRESS	
MY SPIRIT	
MY MIND	

Mood Check-in

Checkmark the box that best describes how you feel.

TODAY	🙂 Happy Content	😐 Blah Neutral	☹️ Sad Sick	😟 Stressed Tired	😠 Angry Annoyed
START OF DAY					
MID-DAY					
END OF DAY					

I NEED: ....

I FEEL THIS WAY BECAUSE: ....
....
....
....

PRAYER FOR THE DAY: ....
....
....
....
....
....

Mindfulness

POSITIVITY

HEY, SIS
YOUR
AWESOMENESS
IS SHOWING!

ELIMINATE
NEGATIVE
SELF-TALK

I AM GRATEFUL FOR:

-
-
-

I will praise thee; for I am fearfully and wonderfully made: marvelous are thy works.
(Psalm 139:14 KJV)

LOOKING FORWARD TO:

....
....
....
....

TO DO:

-
-
-

SAY IT LOUD, I AM...

-
-
-

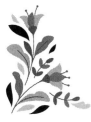
I'm Just Sayin'
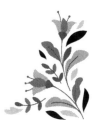

Wellness Tracker
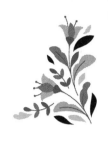

Date: ....

FOCUS	HOW I'M SHOWING UP FOR MYSELF
NUTRITION	
HYDRATION	
EXERCISE	
SLEEP	
DE-STRESS	
MY SPIRIT	
MY MIND	

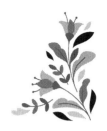

Mood Check-in

Checkmark the box that best describes how you feel.

TODAY	🙂 Happy Content	😐 Blah Neutral	🙁 Sad Sick	😟 Stressed Tired	😠 Angry Annoyed
START OF DAY					
MID-DAY					
END OF DAY					

I NEED: ....

I FEEL THIS WAY BECAUSE: ....
....
....
....

PRAYER FOR THE DAY: ....
....
....
....
....
....

51

Mindfulness

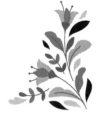

POSITIVITY

I AM GRATEFUL FOR:

-
-
-
-

STAY FOCUSED.

ALWAYS REMEMBER YOUR WHY.

> Beloved, I wish above all things that thou mayest prosper and be in health, even as thy soul prospereth. (3 John 1:2 KJV)

LOOKING FORWARD TO:

....
....
....
....

ELIMINATE NEGATIVE SELF-TALK

TO DO:

-
-
-
-

SAY IT LOUD, I AM...

-
-
-
-

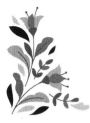

I'm Just Sayin'

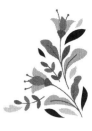

Wellness Tracker

Date: ....

FOCUS	HOW I'M SHOWING UP FOR MYSELF
NUTRITION	
HYDRATION	
EXERCISE	
SLEEP	
DE-STRESS	
MY SPIRIT	
MY MIND	

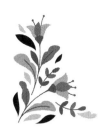
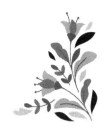

Mood Check-in

Checkmark the box that best describes how you feel.

TODAY	😊 Happy Content	😐 Blah Neutral	🙁 Sad Sick	😟 Stressed Tired	😠 Angry Annoyed
START OF DAY					
MID-DAY					
END OF DAY					

I NEED: ....

I FEEL THIS WAY BECAUSE: ....
....
....
....

PRAYER FOR THE DAY: ....
....
....
....
....
....

Mindfulness

POSITIVITY

I AM GRATEFUL FOR:
-
-
-
-

YOU ARE STONGER, WISER, & BETTER THAN BEFORE.

> In the day when I cried thou answeredst me, and strengthenedst me with strength in my soul.
> (Psalm 138:3 KJV)

LOOKING FORWARD TO:
....
....
....
....

ELIMINATE NEGATIVE SELF-TALK

TO DO:
-
-
-
-

SAY IT LOUD, I AM...
-
-
-
-

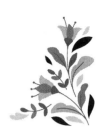

I'm Just Sayin'

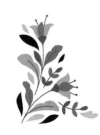
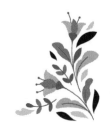

Wellness Tracker

Date: ....

FOCUS	HOW I'M SHOWING UP FOR MYSELF
NUTRITION	
HYDRATION	
EXERCISE	
SLEEP	
DE-STRESS	
MY SPIRIT	
MY MIND	

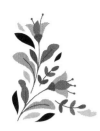
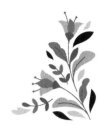

Mood Check-in

Checkmark the box that best describes how you feel.

TODAY	🙂 Happy Content	😐 Blah Neutral	🙁 Sad Sick	Stressed Tired	😠 Angry Annoyed
START OF DAY					
MID-DAY					
END OF DAY					

I NEED: ....

I FEEL THIS WAY BECAUSE: ....
....
....
....

PRAYER FOR THE DAY: ....
....
....
....
....
....

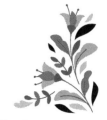

Mindfulness

POSITIVITY

I AM GRATEFUL FOR:

-
-
-

NOPE, RUNNING AWAY FROM EXERCISE DOES NOT COUNT AS CARDIO.

> *Your body is the temple of the Holy Ghost...glorify God in your body, and in your spirit, which are God's. (1 Corinthians 6:19-20)*

LOOKING FORWARD TO:

....
....
....
....

ELIMINATE NEGATIVE SELF-TALK

TO DO:

-
-
-

SAY IT LOUD, I AM...

-
-
-

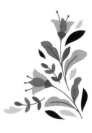

I'm Just Sayin'

Wellness Tracker

Date: ....

FOCUS	HOW I'M SHOWING UP FOR MYSELF
NUTRITION	
HYDRATION	
EXERCISE	
SLEEP	
DE-STRESS	
MY SPIRIT	
MY MIND	

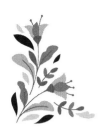
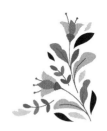

Mood Check-in

Checkmark the box that best describes how you feel.

TODAY	🙂 Happy Content	😐 Blah Neutral	🙁 Sad Sick	😟 Stressed Tired	😠 Angry Annoyed
START OF DAY					
MID-DAY					
END OF DAY					

I NEED: ....

I FEEL THIS WAY BECAUSE: ....
....
....
....

PRAYER FOR THE DAY: ....
....
....
....
....
....

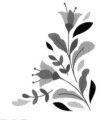

Mindfulness

POSITIVITY

LOOK AT YOU SLAYIN' YOUR GOALS! I SEE YOU, GIRL...I SEE YOU! #LIKEABOSS

I AM GRATEFUL FOR:

-
-
-
-

Commit your actions to the Lord, and your plans will succeed.
(Proverbs 16:3 NLT)

LOOKING FORWARD TO:

....
....
....
....

ELIMINATE NEGATIVE SELF-TALK

TO DO:

-
-
-
-

SAY IT LOUD, I AM...

-
-
-
-

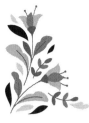

I'm Just Sayin'

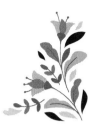

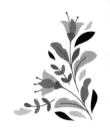

This Week

What mindset do you want to begin the week with?

- o Realistic
- o Honest
- o Fair
- o This is gonna be great!
- o I can't wait to tell everyone about my progress!
- o Diligent & Consistent
- o Eh, we'll see what happens.
- o Maybe this'll work. Won't know until I try.
- o This probably won't work.
- o Negativity will NOT live here, in Jesus' name!
- o Other (in your own words): ....
   ....
   ....

What are your intensions and expectations for this week?

....
....
....
....
....
....
....
....
....
....
....
....

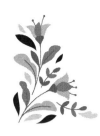
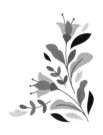

Mindset Matters

Your mindset will play a crucial part in your success. How will you apply this week's mindset to the following?

Mental Health ....
....

Physical Health ....
....

Spiritual Health ....
....

Emotional Health ....
....

Financial Health ....
....

Social Health ....
....

Environmental Health ....
....

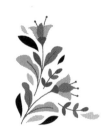

Wellness Tracker

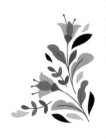

Date: ....

FOCUS	HOW I'M SHOWING UP FOR MYSELF
NUTRITION	
HYDRATION	
EXERCISE	
SLEEP	
DE-STRESS	
MY SPIRIT	
MY MIND	

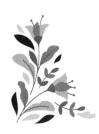
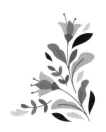

Mood Check-in

Checkmark the box that best describes how you feel.

TODAY	🙂 Happy Content	😐 Blah Neutral	☹️ Sad Sick	😟 Stressed Tired	😠 Angry Annoyed
START OF DAY					
MID-DAY					
END OF DAY					

I NEED: ....

I FEEL THIS WAY BECAUSE: ....
....
....
....

PRAYER FOR THE DAY: ....
....
....
....
....
....

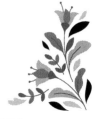

Mindfulness

POSITIVITY

CELEBRATE YOUR WINS. WHAT GETS CELEBRATED GETS REPLICATED!

ELIMINATE NEGATIVE SELF-TALK

I AM GRATEFUL FOR:
-
-
-
-

> Now thanks be unto God, which always causeth us to triumph in Christ.
> (2 Corinthians 2:14 KJV)

LOOKING FORWARD TO:

....
....
....
....

TO DO:
-
-
-
-

SAY IT LOUD, I AM...
-
-
-
-

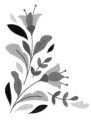

I'm Just Sayin'

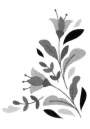

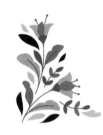

Wellness Tracker

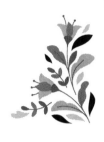

Date: ....

FOCUS	HOW I'M SHOWING UP FOR MYSELF
NUTRITION	
HYDRATION	
EXERCISE	
SLEEP	
DE-STRESS	
MY SPIRIT	
MY MIND	

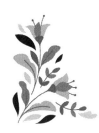
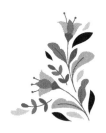

Mood Check-in

Checkmark the box that best describes how you feel.

TODAY	🙂 Happy Content	😐 Blah Neutral	🙁 Sad Sick	😟 Stressed Tired	😠 Angry Annoyed
START OF DAY					
MID-DAY					
END OF DAY					

I NEED: ....

I FEEL THIS WAY BECAUSE: ....
....
....
....

PRAYER FOR THE DAY: ....
....
....
....
....
....

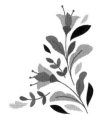

Mindfulness

POSITIVITY

BE LIKE A POSTAGE STAMP.

STICK TO A THING UNTIL YOU GET THERE.

ELIMINATE NEGATIVE SELF-TALK

I AM GRATEFUL FOR:

-
-
-

For when your endurance is fully developed, you will be perfect and complete, needing nothing.
(James 1:4 NLT)

LOOKING FORWARD TO:

....
....
....
....

TO DO:

-
-
-

SAY IT LOUD, I AM...

-
-
-

I'm Just Sayin'
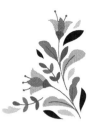

Wellness Tracker

Date: ....

FOCUS	HOW I'M SHOWING UP FOR MYSELF
NUTRITION	
HYDRATION	
EXERCISE	
SLEEP	
DE-STRESS	
MY SPIRIT	
MY MIND	

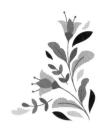

Mood Check-in

Checkmark the box that best describes how you feel.

TODAY	🙂 Happy Content	😐 Blah Neutral	🙁 Sad Sick	😟 Stressed Tired	😠 Angry Annoyed
START OF DAY					
MID-DAY					
END OF DAY					

I NEED: ....

I FEEL THIS WAY BECAUSE: ....
....
....
....

PRAYER FOR THE DAY: ....
....
....
....
....
....

Mindfulness

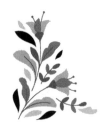
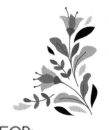

POSITIVITY

I AM GRATEFUL FOR:

-
-
-

BREATHE
(VERB)

TO TAKE IN
LIFE, THEN
REALEASE
IT'S BURDENS.

> *Give all your worries and
> cares to God, for he cares
> about you.*
> *(1 Peter 5:7 NLT)*

LOOKING FORWARD TO:

....
....
....
....

ELIMINATE
NEGATIVE
SELF-TALK

TO DO:

-
-
-
-

SAY IT LOUD, I AM...

-
-
-
-

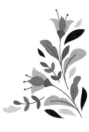

I'm Just Sayin'

 # Wellness Tracker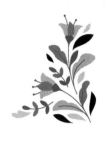

Date: ....

FOCUS	HOW I'M SHOWING UP FOR MYSELF
NUTRITION	
HYDRATION	
EXERCISE	
SLEEP	
DE-STRESS	
MY SPIRIT	
MY MIND	

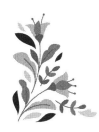 # Mood Check-in

Checkmark the box that best describes how you feel.

TODAY	🙂 Happy Content	😐 Blah Neutral	🙁 Sad Sick	😟 Stressed Tired	😠 Angry Annoyed
START OF DAY					
MID-DAY					
END OF DAY					

I NEED: ....

I FEEL THIS WAY BECAUSE: ....

....

....

....

PRAYER FOR THE DAY: ....

....

....

....

....

....

Mindfulness

POSITIVITY

YOU ARE STRONG & RESILIENT WITH UNLIMITED POTENTIAL.

ELIMINATE NEGATIVE SELF-TALK

I AM GRATEFUL FOR:

-
-
-
-

I can do all things through Christ which strengtheneth me.
(Phillipians 4:13 KJV)

LOOKING FORWARD TO:

....
....
....
....

TO DO:

-
-
-
-

SAY IT LOUD, I AM...

-
-
-
-

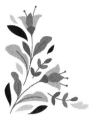
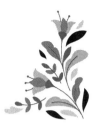

I'm Just Sayin'

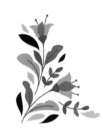

Wellness Tracker

Date: ....

FOCUS	HOW I'M SHOWING UP FOR MYSELF
NUTRITION	
HYDRATION	
EXERCISE	
SLEEP	
DE-STRESS	
MY SPIRIT	
MY MIND	

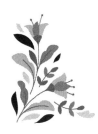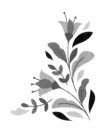

Mood Check-in

Checkmark the box that best describes how you feel.

TODAY	🙂 Happy Content	😐 Blah Neutral	☹️ Sad Sick	😟 Stressed Tired	😠 Angry Annoyed
START OF DAY					
MID-DAY					
END OF DAY					

I NEED: ....

I FEEL THIS WAY BECAUSE: ....
....
....
....

PRAYER FOR THE DAY: ....
....
....
....
....
....

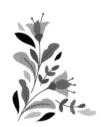

Mindfulness

POSITIVITY

YOU'RE SHOWING UP FOR YOURSELF.

I'M SO PROUD OF YOU!

ELIMINATE NEGATIVE SELF-TALK

I AM GRATEFUL FOR:

-
-
-

So encourage each other and build each other up, just as you are already doing. (1 Thessalonians 5:11 NLT)

LOOKING FORWARD TO:

....
....
....
....

TO DO:

-
-
-

SAY IT LOUD, I AM...

-
-
-

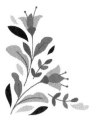
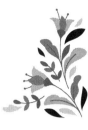

I'm Just Sayin'

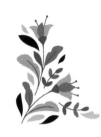 *Wellness Tracker*

Date: ....

FOCUS	HOW I'M SHOWING UP FOR MYSELF
NUTRITION	
HYDRATION	
EXERCISE	
SLEEP	
DE-STRESS	
MY SPIRIT	
MY MIND	

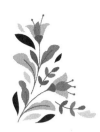
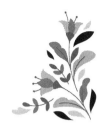

Mood Check-in

Checkmark the box that best describes how you feel.

TODAY	🙂 Happy Content	😐 Blah Neutral	🙁 Sad Sick	😟 Stressed Tired	😠 Angry Annoyed
START OF DAY					
MID-DAY					
END OF DAY					

I NEED: ....

I FEEL THIS WAY BECAUSE: ....
....
....
....

PRAYER FOR THE DAY: ....
....
....
....
....
....

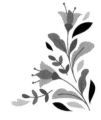

Mindfulness

POSITIVITY

I AM GRATEFUL FOR:

-
-
-

YOUR FUTURE-SELF WILL THANK YOU!

> For I will restore health unto thee, and I will heal thee of thy wounds, saith the LORD.
> (Jeremiah 30:17 KJV)

LOOKING FORWARD TO:

....
....
....
....

ELIMINATE NEGATIVE SELF-TALK

TO DO:

-
-
-

SAY IT LOUD, I AM...

-
-
-

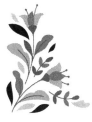
I'm Just Sayin'
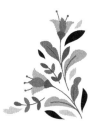

Wellness Tracker

Date: ....

FOCUS	HOW I'M SHOWING UP FOR MYSELF
NUTRITION	
HYDRATION	
EXERCISE	
SLEEP	
DE-STRESS	
MY SPIRIT	
MY MIND	

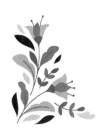

Mood Check-in

Checkmark the box that best describes how you feel.

TODAY	🙂 Happy Content	😐 Blah Neutral	🙁 Sad Sick	😟 Stressed Tired	😠 Angry Annoyed
START OF DAY					
MID-DAY					
END OF DAY					

I NEED: ....

I FEEL THIS WAY BECAUSE: ....
....
....
....

PRAYER FOR THE DAY: ....
....
....
....
....

 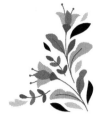

Mindfulness

POSITIVITY

I AM GRATEFUL FOR:

-
-
-

SHE
BELIEVED
SHE COULD,
SO SHE DID.

> Anything is possible if a
> person believes.
> (Mark 9:23 NLT)

LOOKING FORWARD TO:

....
....
....
....

ELIMINATE
NEGATIVE
SELF-TALK

TO DO:

-
-
-

SAY IT LOUD, I AM...

-
-
-
-

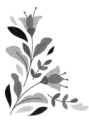

I'm Just Sayin'

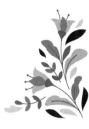

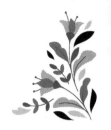

You Did It!

You should be extremely proud of yourself for achieving your 21-day goal. I knew you would show up for yourself because you're AHHH-MAZING!

**** TAKE TIME TO THANK GOD & HAVE A PRAISE BREAK****

HOW WILL YOU CELEBRATE? ....
....
....
....

WHO WILL CELEBRATE WITH YOU?
-
-
-
-

WHAT WAS YOUR FAVORITE PART OF THE JOURNEY?
....
....
....

WHAT WAS YOUR LEAST FAVORITE PART OF THE JOURNEY?
....
....
....

KEEP UP THE GREAT WORK!

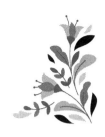

Growth

What have you learned from this experience?

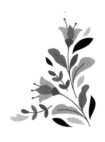

Changes?

What worked and what did not work?

....
....
....
....
....
....
....
....
....
....
....
....
....
....

What will you do different from now on?

....
....
....
....
....
....
....
....
....
....
....
....

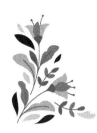
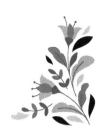

What's Next?

Write the Vision: Do you have a new wellness goal in mind? If so, write out your goal and action plan.

....

....

....

....

....

....

....

....

....

....

....

....

....

....

....

....

....

....

....

....

....

....

....

....

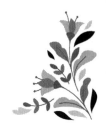

Follow-up

Date: _____

Have you visited your doctor for a check-up? If so, what'd doc think of your progress? ....
....

Are you still applying the things you learned in the first 21 days? If so, how are things going? If not, what happened?
....
....
....
....
....
....
....
....
....
....
....
....
....

Any setbacks? If so, what can you do to get back on track without further delay? ....
....
....
....
....

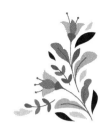

Follow-up

Date: _____

Have you visited your doctor for a check-up? If so, what'd doc think of your progress? ....
....

Are you still applying the things you learned in the first 21 days? If so, how are things going? If not, what happened?
....
....
....
....
....
....
....
....
....
....
....
....

Any setbacks? If so, what can you do to get back on track without further delay? ....
....
....
....
....

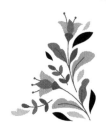

Follow-up

Date: _____

Have you visited your doctor for a check-up? If so, what'd doc think of your progress? ....
....

Are you still applying the things you learned in the first 21 days? If so, how are things going? If not, what happened?
....
....
....
....
....
....
....
....
....
....
....
....
....

Any setbacks? If so, what can you do to get back on track without further delay? ....
....
....
....
....

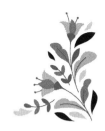

Follow-up

Date: _____

Have you visited your doctor for a check-up? If so, what'd doc think of your progress? ....
....

Are you still applying the things you learned in the first 21 days? If so, how are things going? If not, what happened?

....
....
....
....
....
....
....
....
....
....
....
....
....

Any setbacks? If so, what can you do to get back on track without further delay? ....
....
....
....
....

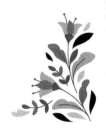

Follow-up

Date: _____

Have you visited your doctor for a check-up? If so, what'd doc think of your progress? ....
....

Are you still applying the things you learned in the first 21 days? If so, how are things going? If not, what happened?
....
....
....
....
....
....
....
....
....
....
....
....
....

Any setbacks? If so, what can you do to get back on track without further delay? ....
....
....
....
....

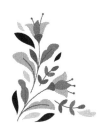

Follow-up

Date: _____

Have you visited your doctor for a check-up? If so, what'd doc think of your progress? ....
....

Are you still applying the things you learned in the first 21 days? If so, how are things going? If not, what happened?
....
....
....
....
....
....
....
....
....
....
....
....
....

Any setbacks? If so, what can you do to get back on track without further delay? ....
....
....
....
....

Follow-up

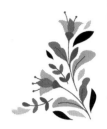

Date: _____

Have you visited your doctor for a check-up? If so, what'd doc think of your progress? ....
....

Are you still applying the things you learned in the first 21 days? If so, how are things going? If not, what happened?
....
....
....
....
....
....
....
....
....
....
....
....
....

Any setbacks? If so, what can you do to get back on track without further delay? ....
....
....
....
....

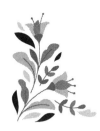
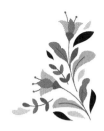

Follow-up

Date: _____

Have you visited your doctor for a check-up? If so, what'd doc think of your progress? ....
....

Are you still applying the things you learned in the first 21 days? If so, how are things going? If not, what happened?

....
....
....
....
....
....
....
....
....
....
....
....
....

Any setbacks? If so, what can you do to get back on track without further delay? ....
....
....
....
....

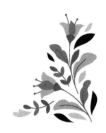

Follow-up

Date: _____

Have you visited your doctor for a check-up? If so, what'd doc think of your progress? ....
....

Are you still applying the things you learned in the first 21 days? If so, how are things going? If not, what happened?

....
....
....
....
....
....
....
....
....
....
....
....
....

Any setbacks? If so, what can you do to get back on track without further delay? ....
....
....
....
....

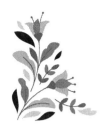
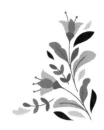

Follow-up

Date: _____

Have you visited your doctor for a check-up? If so, what'd doc think of your progress? ....
....

Are you still applying the things you learned in the first 21 days? If so, how are things going? If not, what happened?
....
....
....
....
....
....
....
....
....
....
....
....
....

Any setbacks? If so, what can you do to get back on track without further delay? ....
....
....
....
....

Notes & Doodles

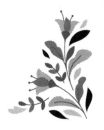

Notes & Doodles

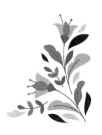

Notes & Doodles

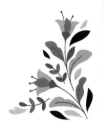

Notes & Doodles

Notes & Doodles

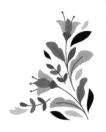

Notes & Doodles

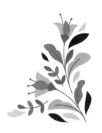

Notes & Doodles

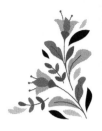

Notes & Doodles

Notes & Doodles

Notes & Doodles

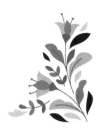

Get In Touch

About PersoNell Wellness

PersoNell Wellness helps women de-stress by losing *weight* of mind, body, spirit, and emotions using personal coaching, journals, and all-natural, handmade self-care products.

"The Weight Is Over!"

Visit www.personellwellness.com for:

- Ordering Additional Products & Services such as scented body butter, sugar scrubs, weight loss coaching, journals, & MORE
- Bulk Order Requests (FOR JOURNALS ONLY)
- Custom Order Requests (FOR JOURNALS ONLY)
- Product Suggestions (FOR JOURNALS ONLY)
- Sharing Your Success Story

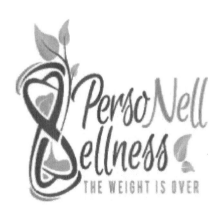

Made in the USA
Middletown, DE
12 December 2022

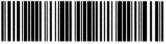

18235807R00068